The Ultimate Keto Diet Cookbook

Lose Weight Fast and Easily Eating Delicious And Healthy
Foods| Gourmet Dinner Recipes

Jane Leaner

Table of Content

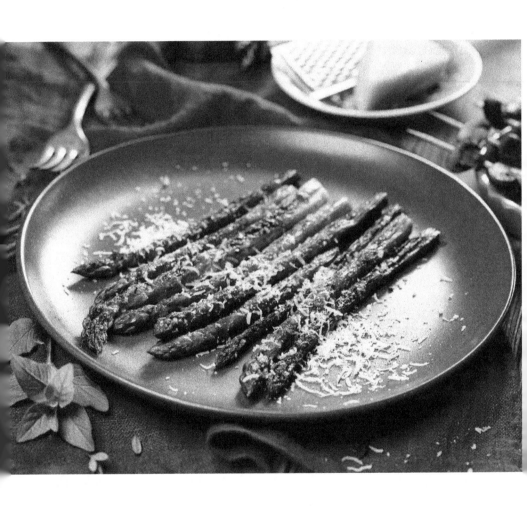

1.   Asparagus & Parmesan

Preparation time: 10 minutes

Cooking time: 6 minutes

Servings: 2

Ingredients:

- 1 teaspoon of sesame oil
- 11 oz. asparagus
- 1 teaspoon chicken stock
- ½ teaspoon ground white pepper
- 3 oz. Parmesan

Directions:

1. Wash the asparagus and chop them roughly.
2. Sprinkle the chopped asparagus with the chicken stock and ground white pepper, then sprinkle the vegetables with the sesame oil and shake them.
3. Place the asparagus in the air fryer's basket and cook the vegetables for 4 minutes at 400 °F.
4. Meanwhile, shred Parmesan cheese.
5. When the time is over, shake the asparagus gently, sprinkle with the shredded cheese and cook the asparagus for 2 minutes more at 400 °F.
6. After this, transfer the cooked asparagus to the serving plates. Enjoy!

Nutrition: Calories 189, Fat 11,6, Fiber 3,4, Carbs 7,9, Protein 17,2.

2.   Avocado Fries

Preparation Time: 10 minutes

Cooking Time: 7 minutes

Servings: 1
Ingredients:

- 1 avocado

- 1/8 tsp. salt

- ¼ cup of panko breadcrumbs

- Bean liquid from a 15-ounce can of white or garbanzo beans

Directions:

1. Peel, pit, and slice up avocado.

2. Take two bowls. In the first bowl, toss salt and breadcrumbs together. Into the second, place the been liquid.

3. Dredge slices of avocado first in the been liquid and then in panko, making sure you are evenly coating.

4. Place coated avocado slices into a single layer in the Air Fryer and cook them for 5 minutes at 390°F.

5. Then, serve with your favorite Keto dipping sauce!

Nutrition: Calories 102, Fat 22, Carbs 1, Protein 9.

3.   Bell-Pepper Corn Wrapped in Tortilla

Preparation Time: 5 minutes

Cooking Time: 15 minutes

Servings: 1
Ingredients:

- ¼ small red bell pepper, chopped

- ¼ small yellow onion, diced

- ¼ tablespoon water

- ½ cobs grilled corn kernels

- 1 large tortilla

- 1 commercial vegan nuggets, chopped

- Mixed greens for garnish

Directions:
1. Preheat the Air Fryer to 400°F.

2. In a skillet heated over medium heat, sauté the vegan nuggets, the onions, bell peppers, and corn kernels and set aside.

3. Place filling inside the corn tortillas and fold the tortillas.

4. Place inside the Air Fryer and cook for 15 minutes until the tortilla wraps are crispy.

—

5. Serve with mixed greens on top and enjoy!

Nutrition: Calories 548, Fat 20,7, Protein 46.

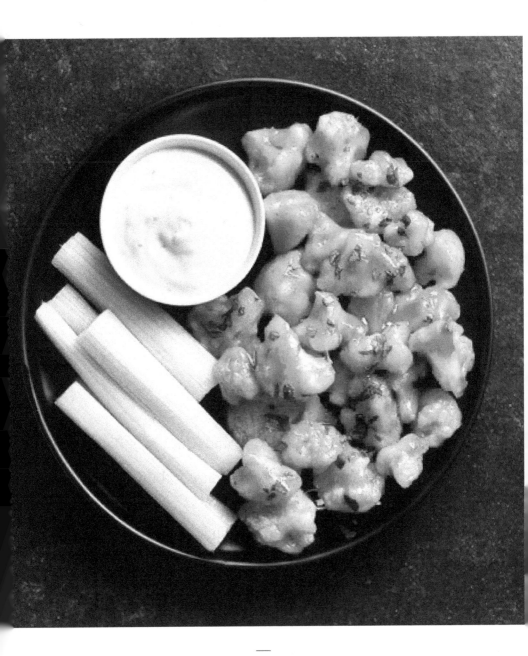

4. Buffalo Cauliflower

Preparation Time: 5 minutes

Cooking Time: 15 minutes

Servings: 1

Ingredients:

- Cauliflower

- 1 cup of panko breadcrumbs

- 1 tsp. salt

- 2 cups of cauliflower florets

- Buffalo coating

- ¼ cup of Vegan Buffalo sauce

- ¼ cup of melted vegan butter

Directions:

1. Melt butter in the microwave and whisk in buffalo sauce.

2. Dip each cauliflower floret into a buffalo mixture, ensuring it gets coated well.

3. Mix breadcrumbs with salt and immerse florets into breadcrumbs.

4. Place them into Air Fryer and cook them for 15 minutes at 350°F. When slightly browned, they are ready to eat!

14

5. Serve with your favorite Keto dipping sauce and enjoy!

Nutrition: Calories 194, Fat 17, Protein 10.

5. Braised Collard Greens in Peanut Sauce with Pork Tenderloin

Preparation Time: 20 minutes

Cooking Time: 1 hour and 15 minutes

Servings: 4

Ingredients:

- 2 cups of chicken stock

- 12 cups of chopped collard greens

- 5 tablespoon of powdered peanut butter

- 3 cloves of garlic, crushed

- 1 teaspoon of salt

- ½ teaspoon of allspice

- ½ teaspoon of black pepper

- 2 teaspoons of lemon juice

- ¾ teaspoon of hot sauce

- 1 ½ lb. of pork tenderloin

Directions:

1. In a saucepan, put the cabbage, garlic, chicken broth, hot sauce, half the pepper, and salt and simmer for about an hour or until the cabbage is tender.

2. Then, stir in the allspice, lemon juice, and powdered peanut butter and set aside warm.

3. Season the pork fillet with the remaining pepper and salt and cook in the oven for 10 minutes. (Turn the fillet every 2 minutes to obtain an even browning).

4. Remove from the oven and leave to rest for about 5 minutes.

5. Slice the pork and serve with the cabbage garnish.

Nutrition: Calories 320, Fat 10, Carbs 15, Protein 45.

6. Carrot Lentil Burgers

Preparation Time: 10 minutes

Cooking Time: 12 minutes

Servings: 2

Ingredients:

- 6 oz. lentils, cooked

- 1 egg

- 2 oz. carrot, grated

- 1 teaspoon semolina

- ½ teaspoon salt

- 1 teaspoon turmeric

- 1 tablespoon butter

Directions:

1. Preheat the air fryer to 360 °F.

2. Into the bowl crack the egg and whisk it.

3. Add the cooked lentils and mash the mixture with the help of the fork.

4. Then sprinkle the mixture with the grated carrot, semolina, salt, and turmeric, mix it up, and make the medium burgers.

5. Put the lentil burgers in the air fryer and cook for 12 minutes.

6. Flip the burgers into another side after 6 minutes of cooking, then chill the cooked lentil burgers and serve them.

Nutrition: Calories 404, Fat 9, Fiber 26,9, Carbs 56, Protein 25,3.

7.   Cauliflower Crust Pizza

Preparation Time: 20 minutes

Cooking Time: 45 minutes

Servings: 4

Ingredients:

- 1 cauliflower (it should be cut into smaller portions)

- ¼ grated parmesan cheese

- 1 egg

- 1 tsp. of Italian seasoning

- ¼ tsp. of kosher salt

- 2 cups of freshly grated mozzarella

- ¼ cup of spicy pizza sauce

- Basil leaves, for garnishing

Directions:

1. Preheating the oven and rim the baking sheet with the parchment paper.

2. Process the cauliflower into a fine powder, and then transfer to a bowl.

3. Put it into the microwave and cook for about 5-6 minutes to get it soft.

4. Transfer the cauliflower to a clean and dry kitchen towel and leave it to cool off.

5. When it is cold, get rid of all the moisture by wringing the towel.

6. Into a bowl, put the cauliflower, Italian seasoning, Parmesan, egg, salt, and mozzarella and stir very well until well combined.

7. Transfer the mixture to the baking sheet previously prepared, pressing it into a 10-inch round shape.

8. Bake for 10-15 minutes until it becomes golden in color.

9. Remove from the oven and top it with the spicy pizza sauce and mozzarella, then bake again for 10 more minutes until the cheese melts.

10. Remove from the oven, garnish using fresh basil leaves and serve!.

Nutrition: Calories 74, Fat 4, Fiber 2, Carbs 4, Protein 6.

8. Cauliflower Shakshuka

Preparation Time: 5 minutes

Cooking Time: 20 minutes

Servings: 2

Ingredients:

- 1 pound of riced cauliflower
- 4 tablespoons of extra virgin olive oil
- 4 tablespoons of chopped onion
- 1 tablespoon of India seasoning (or ground mustard, ground coriander, cumin, garlic, cayenne, turmeric, natural sea salt)
- 1 1/5 -ounce diced tomatoes (with no added sugar)
- 1 1/5 -ounce pureed tomatoes (with no added sugar)
- 4 fresh eggs
- Fresh parsley for garnish (optional)

Directions:

1. Cook the cauliflower following the instructions on the package.

2. In a skillet, add the oil and heat it over medium-high heat.

3. Stir in the onions and saute for about 2 minutes or until translucent.

4. Sprinkle the mixture with the spices and brown for another minute.

5. Add the cooked cauliflower to the pan, mix thoroughly, and season with salt.

6. Incorporate the tomatoes and mix well.

7. Cover the pan and bring the mixture to a boil, then simmer for another 5 minutes.

8. Open the pot, break the eggs into the mixture, and season with pepper and salt.

9. Close the pan and cook for 3 minutes to poach the egg or cook for about 6-7 for a hard-cooked egg.

10. Turn off the heat, garnish with fresh parsley and serve.

Nutrition: Calories 228, Fat 14,5, Fiber 3,6, Carbs 10,3, Protein 15,3.

9. Cheddar Potato Gratin

Preparation Time: 15 minutes

Cooking Time: 20 minutes

Servings: 2

Ingredients:

- 2 potatoes

- 1/3 cup half and half

- 1 tablespoon oatmeal flour

- ¼ teaspoon ground black pepper

- 1 egg

- 2 oz. Cheddar cheese

Directions:

1. Preheat the air fryer to 365 °F.

2. Wash the potatoes, slice them into thin pieces, and put them into an air fryer for 10 minutes.

3. Meanwhile, combine the half and half, oatmeal flour, and ground black pepper, crack the egg and whisk it carefully, then shred the cheddar cheese.

4. When the potato is cooked, take 2 ramekins and place the potatoes on them and pour the mixture.

5. Sprinkle the gratin with shredded Cheddar cheese, put the gratin into the oven, and cook it for 10 minutes at 360 °F.

6. Serve the meal immediately. Enjoy!

Nutrition: Calories 353, Fat 16,6, Fiber 5,4, Carbs 37,2, Protein 15.

10. Cheddar Portobello Mushrooms

Preparation Time: 15 minutes

Cooking Time: 6 minutes

Servings: 2

Ingredients:

- 2 Portobello mushroom hats

- 2 slices Cheddar cheese

- ¼ cup panko breadcrumbs

- ½ teaspoon salt

- ½ teaspoon ground black pepper

- 1 egg

- 1 teaspoon of oatmeal

- 2 oz. bacon, chopped cooked

Directions:

1. Preheat the air fryer to 400 °F.

2. Into a bowl, crack the egg and whisk it.

3. Into another bowl, combine the ground black pepper, oatmeal, salt, and breadcrumbs.

4. Dip the mushroom hats in the whisked egg and then, coat the mushroom hats in the breadcrumb mixture.

5. Place the mushrooms in the air fryer basket tray and cook for 3 minutes.

6. After this, put the chopped bacon and sliced cheese over the mushroom hats, and cook the meal for 3 minutes.

7. Let it chill before serving and enjoy them!

Nutrition: Calories 376, Fat 24,1, Fiber 1,8, Carbs 14,6, Protein 25,2.

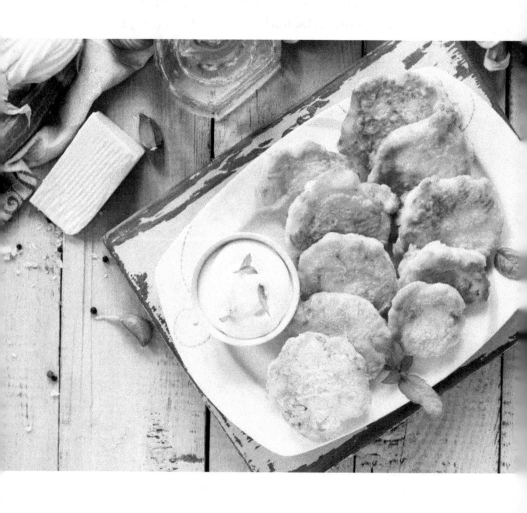

11.   Cheesy Cauliflower Fritters

Preparation Time: 10 minutes

Cooking Time: 7 minutes

Servings: 1

Ingredients:

- ½ cup of chopped parsley

- 1 cup of Italian breadcrumbs

- 1/3 cup of shredded mozzarella cheese

- 1/3 cup of shredded sharp cheddar cheese

- 1 egg

- 2 minced garlic cloves

- 3 chopped scallions

- 1 head of cauliflower

Directions:

1. Cut the cauliflower up into florets, wash it well, and pat dry.

2. Place cauliflower into a food processor and pulse 20-30 seconds till it looks like rice.

3. Place the cauliflower rice into a bowl and mix with pepper, salt, egg, cheese, breadcrumbs, garlic, and scallions.

4. With hands, form 15 patties, adding more breadcrumbs if needed.

5. Cook them into the oven for 14 minutes at 390 °F, and flopping patties after half cook.

6. Serve and enjoy!

Nutrition: Calories 209, Fat 17, Carbs 0,5, Protein 6.

12. Coconut Battered Cauliflower Bites

Preparation Time: 5 minutes

Cooking Time: 20 minutes

Servings: 1

Ingredients:

- Salt and pepper to taste

- 1 flax egg or one tablespoon flaxseed meal + 3 tablespoon water

- 1 small cauliflower, cut into florets

- 1 teaspoon of mixed spice

- ½ teaspoon of mustard powder

- 2 tablespoons maple syrup

- 1 clove of garlic, minced

- 2 tablespoons soy sauce

- 1/3 cup oats flour

- 1/3 cup plain flour

- 1/3 cup desiccated coconut

Directions:

1. In a mixing bowl, mix oats, flour, and desiccated coconut and season with salt and pepper to taste, then set aside.

2. In another bowl, place the flax egg, add a pinch of salt to taste, and set aside.

3. Season the cauliflower with mixed spice and mustard powder.

4. Dip the florets in the flax egg first, then in the flour mixture.

5. Place it into an Air Fryer and cook at 400°F for 15 minutes.

6. Meanwhile, place the maple syrup, garlic, and soy sauce in a saucepan and heat over medium flame. When it boils, adjust the heat to low until the sauce thickens.

7. When florets are cooked, place them in the saucepan with the sauce and toss well. Then, place inside Air Fryer and cook them for another 5 minutes. Serve and enjoy!

Nutrition: Calories 154, Fat 2,3, Protein 4,7.

13.   Corn on Cobs

Preparation Time: 10 minutes

Cooking Time: 10 minutes

Servings: 2

Ingredients:

- 2 fresh corn on cobs

- 2 teaspoon butter

- 1 teaspoon salt

- 1 teaspoon paprika

- ¼ teaspoon olive oil

Directions:

1. Preheat the air fryer to 400°F.

2. Seasoning the corn on cobs with salt, paprika, and olive oil.

3. Place the corn on cobs in the air fryer's basket and cook them for 10 minutes.

4. When the time is over, transfer the corn on cobs to the serving plates, rub with the butter gently and serve immediately.

Nutrition: Calories 122, Fat 5,5, Fiber 2,4, Carbs 17,6, Protein 3,2.

---

14.   Cremini Mushroom Satay

Preparation Time: 10 minutes

Cooking Time: 6 minutes

Servings: 2

Ingredients:

- 7 oz. cremini mushrooms

- 2 tablespoon coconut milk

- 1 tablespoon butter

- 1 teaspoon chili flakes

- ½ teaspoon balsamic vinegar

- ½ teaspoon curry powder

- ½ teaspoon white pepper

Directions:

1. Wash the mushrooms carefully and then sprinkle them with chili flakes, curry powder, and white pepper.

2. Preheat the air fryer to 400 °F.

3. Put the butter in the air fryer basket and melt it.

4. Put the mushrooms in the air fryer and cook for 2 minutes.

5. Shake the mushrooms well and sprinkle with the coconut milk and balsamic vinegar, then cook the mushrooms for 4 minutes more at 400 °F.

6. Skewer the mushrooms on the wooden sticks, serve and enjoy!

Nutrition: Calories 116, Fat 9,5, Fiber 1,3, Carbs 5,6, Protein 3.

15. Crispy Jalapeno Coins

Preparation Time: 10 minutes

Cooking Time: 5 minutes

Servings: 1

Ingredients:

- 1 egg

- 2/3 tbsp. coconut flour

- 1sliced and seeded jalapeno

- Pinch of garlic powder

- Pinch of onion powder

- Bit of Cajun seasoning (optional)

- Pinch of pepper and salt

Directions:

1. Preheated Air Fryer to 400 degrees.

2. Mix all dry ingredients.

3. Pat jalapeno slices dry. Dip them into the egg wash and then into the dry mixture.

4. Put coated jalapeno slices in Air Fryer in a singular layer and spray them with olive oil.

---

5. Lock the air fryer lid. Set temperature to 350°F and set time to 5 minutes. Cook just till crispy, then serve and enjoy!

Nutrition: Calories 128, Fat 8, Protein 7.

16.   Crispy Roasted Broccoli

Preparation Time: 10 minutes

Cooking Time: 8 minutes

Servings: 1
Ingredients:

- ¼ tsp. Masala

- ½ tsp. red chili powder

- ½ tsp. salt

- ¼ tsp. turmeric powder

- 1 tbsp. chickpea flour

- 1 tbsp. yogurt

- ½ pound broccoli

Directions:
1. Preheat the air fryer to 390 degrees.

2. Cut the broccoli into florets and immerse them into a bowl of water with two teaspoons of salt for at least half an hour to remove impurities.

3. Remove the broccoli florets from the water and let them drain.

4. Mix all the other ingredients to create a marinade.

5. Stir the broccoli flowers into the marinade and let them rest for 15-30 minutes.

6. Place the marinated broccoli flowers in the deep fryer and cook for 10 minutes at 350 ° F. Serve and enjoy.

Nutrition: Calories 96, Fat 1,3, Carbs 4,5, Protein 7.

17.   Crispy Rye Bread Snacks with Guacamole and Anchovies

Preparation Time: 10 minutes

Cooking Time: 10 minutes

Servings: 4

Ingredients:

- 4 slices of rye bread

- Guacamole

- Anchovies in oil

Directions:

1. Cut each slice of bread into three strips of bread.

2. Place in the basket of the air fryer, a little at a time, and cook for 10 minutes at 180°C.

3. When all the strips of rye bread are crispy, put a layer of guacamole (homemade or commercial), and two anchovies on the top.

4. Serve and enjoy!

Nutrition: Calories 180, Fat 11, Fiber 0,9, Carbs 4, Protein 4.

18.   Crispy-Topped Baked Vegetables

Preparation Time: 10 minutes

Cooking Time: 40 minutes

Servings: 4
Ingredients:
- 2 tbsp. oof live oil

- 1 onion, chopped

- 1 celery stalk, chopped

- 2 carrots, grated

- ½ pound turnips, sliced

- 1 cup of vegetable broth

- 1 tsp. turmeric

- Sea salt and black pepper, to taste

- ½ tsp. of liquid smoke

- 1 cup of Parmesan cheese, shredded

- 2 tbsp of fresh chives, chopped

Directions:
1. Preheat the oven to 360 °F and grease a baking sheet with olive oil.

2. Put a little oil in a pan and heat over medium heat.

3. Add the onion and sauté until soft. Then add it to the turnips, carrots, and celery and cook for 4 minutes.

4. Remove the vegetables and place them in the already oiled baking tray.

5. Combine the vegetable stock with turmeric, pepper, liquid smoke, and salt and distribute this mixture over the vegetables.

6. Sprinkle with Parmesan cheese and bake for about 30 minutes.

7. Remove from the oven, garnish with chives, and serve.

Nutrition: Calories 242, Fat 16,3, Carbs 6,8, Protein 16,3.

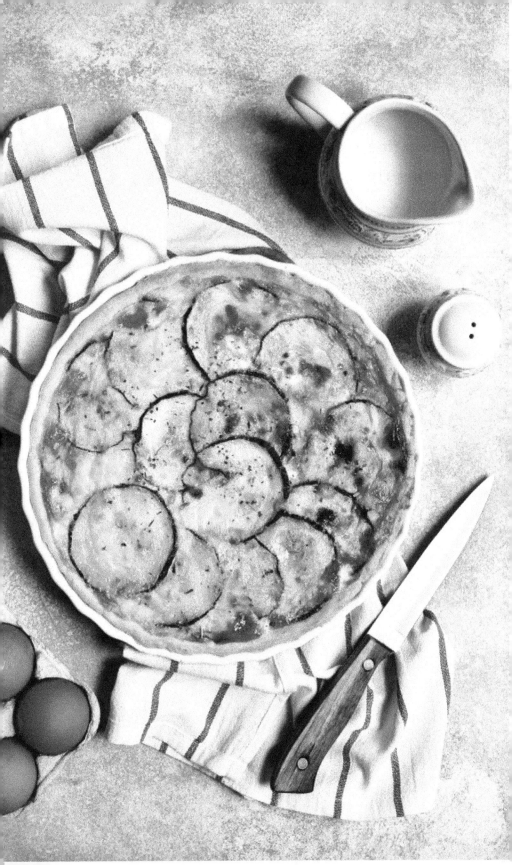

19.   Delicious Zucchini Quiche

Preparation Time: 15 minutes

Cooking Time: 1 hour

Servings: 8

Ingredients:

- 6 eggs

- 2 medium zucchinis, shredded

- ½ tsp. of dried basil

- 2 garlic cloves, minced

- 1 tbsp. dry onion, minced

- 2 tbsp. parmesan cheese, grated

- 2 tbsp. fresh parsley, chopped

- ½ cup of olive oil

- 1 cup of cheddar cheese, shredded

- ¼ cup of coconut flour

- 3/4 cup almond flour

- ½ tsp. salt

Directions:

1. Preheat the oven to 350 degrees, grease the 9-inch pan and set aside.

2. Squeeze the excess liquid from the zucchini.

3. Add all the ingredients to the large bowl and mix until smooth, then pour into the prepared pan.

4. Bake in a preheated oven for 45-60 minutes, then remove from the oven, allow to cool completely, slice, and serve.

Nutrition: Calories 288, Fat 26,3, Carbs 5, Protein 11.

20. Eggplant Ratatouille

Preparation Time: 15 minutes

Cooking Time: 15 minutes

Servings: 2

Ingredients:

- 1 Eggplant

- 1 sweet yellow pepper

- 3 cherry tomatoes

- 1/3 white onion, chopped

- ½ teaspoon garlic clove, sliced

- 1 teaspoon olive oil

- ½ teaspoon ground black pepper

- ½ teaspoon Italian seasoning

Directions:

1. Preheat the air fryer to 360 °F.

2. Peel and chop the eggplants; the cherry tomatoes and onion, the sweet yellow pepper, and garlic.

3. Season with olive oil, ground black pepper, and Italian seasoning.

4. Add all chopped vegetables to the air fryer basket.

5. Shake the vegetables gently and cook for 15 minutes. Stir them after 8 minutes of cooking.

6. Transfer the cooked ratatouille to the serving plates and enjoy!

Nutrition: Calories 149, Fat 3,7, Fiber 11,7, Carbs 28,9, Protein 5,1.

21.   Fried Avocado

Preparation Time: 15 minutes

Cooking Time: 10 minutes

Servings: 2

Ingredients:

- 2 avocados cut into wedges 25 mm. thick

- 50 g. breadcrumbs

- 2 g. garlic powder

- 2 g. onion powder

- 1 g. smoked paprika

- 1 g. cayenne pepper

- Salt and pepper to taste

- 60 g. all-purpose flour

- 2 eggs, beaten

- Nonstick spray oil

- Tomato sauce or ranch sauce, to serve

Directions:

1. Preheat the air fryer.

2. Cut the avocados into 25 mm. thick pieces.

3. Into a bowl, combine the crumbs, garlic powder, onion powder, smoked paprika, cayenne pepper, and salt.

4. Dip each wedge of avocado in the flour, then dip in the beaten eggs and stir in the breadcrumb mixture.

5. Place the avocados in the preheated air fryer baskets, spray with oil spray, and cook at 205°C for 10 minutes.

6. Turn the fried avocado halfway through cooking and sprinkle with cooking oil.

7. Serve with tomato sauce or ranch sauce. Enjoy!

Nutrition: Calories 123, Fat 11, Fiber 0, Carbs 2, Protein 4.

22.   Fried Zucchini

Preparation Time: 10 minutes

Cooking Time: 8 minutes

Servings: 4

Ingredients:

- 2 medium zucchinis, cut into strips 19 mm. thick

- 60 g all-purpose flour

- 12 g of salt

- 2 g black pepper

- 2 beaten eggs

- 15 ml. of milk

- 80 g Italian seasoned breadcrumbs

- 25 g grated Parmesan cheese

- Nonstick spray oil

- Ranch sauce, to serve

Directions:

1. Preheat the air fryer, set it to 175°C.

2. Cut the zucchini into strips 19 mm thick.

3. Mix the flour, salt, and pepper on a plate and mix the eggs and milk into a bowl.

4. In another dish, mix breadcrumbs, and Parmesan cheese.

5. Cover each piece of zucchini before with flour, then dip them in egg and milk mixture, and finally pass them through the crumbs. Then leave aside.

6. Place the covered zucchini in the preheated air fryer and spray with oil spray. Cook them for 8 minutes.

7. Serve with tomato sauce or ranch sauce.

Nutrition: Calories 68, Fat 11, Fiber 143, Carbs 2, Protein 4.

23.   Green Pea Guacamole

Preparation Time: 15 minutes

Cooking Time: 35 minutes

Servings: 4

Ingredients:

- 1 teaspoon of crushed garlic

- 1 chopped tomato

- 3 cups of frozen green peas (chopped)

- 5 green chopped onions

- 1/6 teaspoon of hot sauce

- ½ teaspoon of grounded cumin

- ½ cup of lime juice

Directions:

1. In a kitchen robot, add the peas, garlic, lime juice, and cumin and blend them until it is smoothened.

2. In the mixture, add the tomatoes, green onion, and hot sauce and stir, then, add salt to taste.

3. Cover it and put it into the refrigerator for a minimum of 30 minutes. This will allow the flavor to blend very well.

4. You can serve the sauce on slices of toast or as you like!

Nutrition: Calories 40,7, Fat 0,2, Fiber 1,7, Carbs 7,6, Protein 2,7.

24.　Grilled Eggplants

Preparation Time: 10 minutes

Cooking Time: 10 minutes

Servings: 4

Ingredients:

- 1 large eggplant, cut into thick circles

- Salt and pepper to taste

- 1 tsp. of smoked paprika

- 1 tbsp.of coconut flour

- 1 tsp. of lime juice

- 1 tbsp. of olive oil

Directions:

1. Coat the eggplants in smoked paprika, salt, pepper, lime juice, coconut flour, and let it sit for 10 minutes.

2. In a grilling pan, add the olive oil and grill the eggplants for 3 minutes on each side, then serve.

Nutrition: Calories 34,5 - Fat 0,1, Fiber 2,4, Carbs 4,8, Protein 0,8.

25. Grilled Mahi-Mahi with Jicama Slaw

Preparation Time: 20 minutes

Cooking Time: 10 minutes

Servings: 4

Ingredients:

- 1 teaspoon each pepper and salt, divided

- 1 tablespoon of lime juice, divided

- 2 tablespoon + 2 teaspoons of extra virgin olive oil

- 4 raw mahi-mahi fillets, which should be about 8 oz. each

- ½ cucumber which should be thinly cut into long strips like matchsticks (it should yield about 1 cup)

- 1 jicama, which should be thinly cut into long strips like matchsticks (it should yield about 3 cups)

- 1 cup of alfalfa sprouts

- 2 cups of coarsely chopped watercress

Directions:

1. In a small bowl, combine ½ teaspoon of both pepper and salt, one teaspoon of lime juice, and two teaspoons of oil.

2. Then brush the mahi-mahi fillets all through with the olive oil mixture.

3. Grill the mahi-mahi on medium-high heat for about 5 minutes per side.

4. Take two bowls. In the first bowl, combine the watercress, cucumber, jicama, and alfalfa sprouts. In the second bowl, combine ½ teaspoon of both pepper and salt, two teaspoons of lime juice, and two tablespoons of extra virgin oil in a small bowl.

5. Pour the contents of the second bowl into the first bowl, and toss together to combine.

6. Serve the Grilled Mahi-Mahi with Jicama Slaw and enjoy!

Nutrition: Calories 320, Fat 11, Carbs 10, Protein 44.

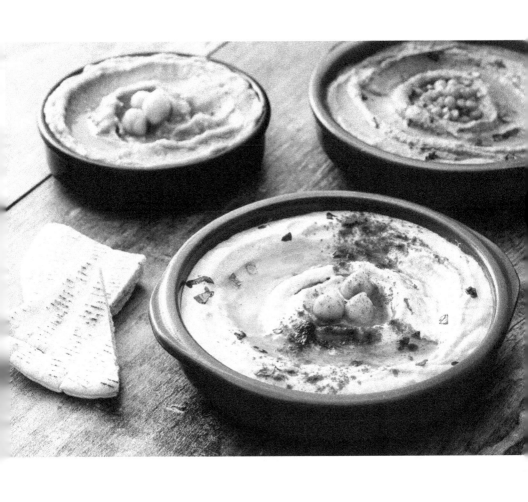

26.   Hummus

Preparation Time: 10 minutes

Cooking Time: 10 minutes

Servings: 10+

Ingredients:

- 4 cups of cooked garbanzo beans
- 1 cup of water
- 1 ½ tablespoon of lemon juice
- 2 teaspoons of ground cumin
- 1 ½ teaspoon of ground coriander.
- 1 teaspoon of finely chopped garlic
- ½ teaspoon of salt
- ¼ teaspoon of fresh ground pepper
- Paprika for garnish

Directions:

1. On a food processor, place together with the garbanzo beans, lemon juice, water, garlic, salt, and pepper and process it until it becomes smooth and creamy (if necessary, add more water).

2. Then spoon out the hummus in a serving bowl, sprinkle with paprika and serve.

Nutrition: Calories 34,5 - Fat 1,7, Fiber 0,6, Carbs 2,5, Protein 0,7.

27.   Jalapeno Cheese Balls

Preparation Time: 10 minutes

Cooking Time: 8 minutes

Servings: 1

Ingredients:

- 1-ounce cream cheese

- 1/6 cup shredded mozzarella cheese

- 1/6 cup shredded Cheddar cheese

- ½ jalapeños, finely chopped

- ½ cup breadcrumbs

- 2 eggs

- ½ cup all-purpose flour

- Salt and pepper

- Cooking oil

Directions:

1. In a medium bowl, combine the cream cheese, mozzarella, Cheddar, and jalapeños and mix well.

2. Form the cheese mixture into balls about an inch thick and put them in a sheet pan.

3. Place the sheet pan in the freezer for 15 minutes. (It will help the cheese balls maintain their shape while frying).

4. Spray the Air Fryer basket with cooking oil.

5. Take three bowls. In the first bowl place the breadcrumbs. In the second bowl, beat the eggs. In the third bowl, combine the flour with salt and pepper to taste, and mix well.

6. Remove the cheese balls from the freezer and plunge them in the flour, then the eggs, and then the breadcrumbs.

7. Place the cheese balls in the Instant Crisp Air Fryer. Spray with cooking oil. Lock the air fryer lid. Cook for 8 minutes.

8. Open the Air Fryer and flip the cheese balls and cook for another 4 minutes.

9. Cool before serving. Enjoy!

Nutrition: Calories 96, Fat 6, Protein 4.

28.   Mixed Potato Gratin

Preparation Time: 20 minutes

Cooking Time: 7 hours

Servings: 8

Ingredients:

- 6 Yukon Gold potatoes, thinly sliced

- 3 sweet potatoes, peeled and thinly sliced

- 2 onions, thinly sliced

- 4 garlic cloves, minced

- 3 tablespoons whole-wheat flour

- 4 cups 2% milk, divided

- 1 ½ cups roasted vegetable broth

- 3 tablespoons melted butter

- 1 teaspoon dried thyme leaves

- 1 ½ cups shredded Havarti cheese

Directions:

1. Grease a 6-quart slow cooker with straight vegetable oil and arrange the potatoes, onions, and garlic in layers.

2. In a large bowl, add the flour with ½ cup of the milk and mix well.

3. Gradually add the remaining milk, stirring with a wire whisk to avoid lumps.

4. Stir in the vegetable broth, melted butter, and thyme leaves.

5. Pour the milk mixture over the potatoes in the slow cooker and top with the cheese.

6. Cover and cook on low for 7 to 9 hours, until the potatoes are tender.

Nutrition: Calories 415, Fat 22, Fiber 3, Carbs 42, Protein 17.

29. Mushroom & Jalapeño Stew

Preparation Time: 20 minutes

Cooking Time: 50 minutes

Servings: 4
Ingredients:

- 2 tsp. of olive oil

- 1 cup of leeks, chopped

- 1 garlic clove, minced

- ½ cup of celery stalks, chopped

- ½ cup o carrots, chopped

- 1 green bell pepper, chopped

- 1 jalapeño pepper, chopped

- 2 ½ cups mushrooms, sliced

- 1 ½ cups vegetable stock

- 2 tomatoes, chopped

- 2 thyme sprigs, chopped

- 1 rosemary sprig chopped

- 2 bay leaves

- ½ tsp. salt

- ¼ tsp. ground black pepper

- 2 tbsp. vinegar

Directions:
1. In a pan pour the oil and heat over medium heat, then, add in garlic and leeks and sauté until soft and translucent.

2. Add in the black pepper, celery, mushrooms, and carrots and cook for 12 minutes stirring occasionally (if necessary, stir in a splash of vegetable stock to ensure there is no sticking).

3. Stir in the rest of the ingredients, set heat to medium, and allow to simmer for 25 to 35 minutes or until cooked through. Serve warm and enjoy!

Nutrition: Calories 65, Fat 2,7, Carbs 9, Protein 2,7.

30. Mushrooms Stuffed with Tomato

Preparation Time: 5 minutes

Cooking Time: 50 minutes

Servings: 4

Ingredients:

- 8 large mushrooms

- 250 g of minced meat

- 4 cloves of garlic

- Extra virgin olive oil

- Salt

- Ground pepper

- Flour, beaten egg, breadcrumbs

- Frying oil

- Fried tomato sauce

Directions:

1. Remove the stem from the mushrooms and chop it.

2. In a pan, put some extra virgin olive oil and add the minced garlic and the mushroom stems and sauté.

3. Add the minced meat and sauté well until the meat is well-cooked. Then season.

———

4. Fill the mushrooms with the minced meat, press well, and take them to the freezer for 30 minutes.

5. Pass the mushrooms with flour, beaten egg, and breadcrumbs and then, place them in the basket of the air fryer.

6. Cook the mushrooms for 20 minutes at 180 °C.

7. Once they're cooked, distribute them in the dishes and serve them with a cover of tomato sauce.

Nutrition: Calories 160, Fat 11, Fiber 0, Carbs 2, Protein 4.

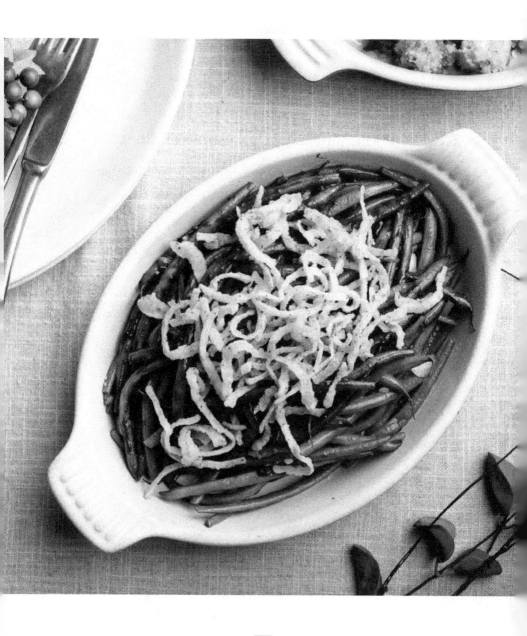

31.   Onion Green Beans

Preparation Time: 10 minutes

Cooking Time: 12 minutes

Servings: 2

Ingredients:

- 11 oz. green beans

- 1 tablespoon onion powder

- 1 tablespoon olive oil

- ½ teaspoon salt

- ¼ teaspoon chili flakes

Directions:

1. Preheat the air fryer to 400 °F.

2. Wash the green beans carefully and place them in the bowl, then sprinkle the green beans with the onion powder, salt, chili flakes, and olive oil and shake the green beans carefully.

3. Put the green beans in the air fryer and cook them for 8 minutes.

4. After this, shake the green beans and cook them for 4 minutes more at 400 F.

5. Once they're cooked, shake the green beans and serve them as the side dish.

Nutrition: Calories 134, Fat 7,2, Fiber 5,5, Carbs 13,9, Protein 3,2.

32.   Pizza Hack

Preparation Time: 5 minutes

Cooking Time: 15 minutes

Servings: 1

Ingredients:

- ¼ fueling of garlic mashed potato

- ½ egg whites

- ¼ tablespoon of baking powder

- 3/4 oz. of reduced-fat shredded mozzarella

- 1/8 cup of sliced white mushrooms

- 1/16 cup of pizza sauce

- 3/4 oz. of ground beef

- ¼ sliced black olives

Directions:

1. Preheating the oven to 400°.

2. Mix your baking powder and garlic potato packet and then add egg whites to your mixture and stir well until it blends.

3. Line the baking sheet with parchment paper and pour the mixed batter onto it.

4. Put another parchment paper on top of the batter and spread out the batter to a 1/8-inch circle. Then place another baking sheet on top; (in this way, the batter is between two baking sheets).

5. Place into an oven and bake for about 8 minutes until the pizza crust is golden brown.

6. Once the crust is baked, remove the top layer of parchment paper carefully.

FOR THE TOPPINGS:

7. Place your ground beef in a sauté pan and fry till it's brown; meanwhile, wash the mushrooms very well.

8. Put the toppings on top of the crust and bake for an extra 8 minutes.

9. Once the pizza is ready, slide it off the parchment paper, put it on a plate, and serve!

Nutrition: Calories 478, Fat 29, Carbs 22, Protein 30.

33. Cloud Bread

Preparation Time: 25 minutes

Cooking Time: 35 minutes

Servings: 3

Ingredients:

- ½ cup of fat-free 0% plain Greek yogurt (4.4 oz)

- 3 eggs, separated

- 16 teaspoons cream of tartar

- 1 packet sweetener (a granulated sweetener just like stevia)

Directions:

1. Place a bowl and a whisk attachment in the freezer for about 30 minutes and preheat your oven to 300 degrees.

2. After 30 minutes, remove the mixing bowl and whisk attachment from the freezer.

3. Separate the eggs and put the egg whites in the cold bowl with the cream of tartar and beat this mixture until the egg whites turn to stiff peaks.

4. In another bowl add the yolks, the sweetener, and yogurt and mix well.

5. Fold this mix carefully into the egg whites with slow movements from the bottom up.

73

6. Place baking paper on a baking tray and spray with cooking spray.

7. Scoop out six equally-sized "blobs" of the "dough" onto the parchment paper and bake them for about 25-35 minutes. (Once they're done as they will get brownish at the top and have some crack). Serve!

Nutrition: Calories 234, Fiber 8, Carbs 5, Protein 23.

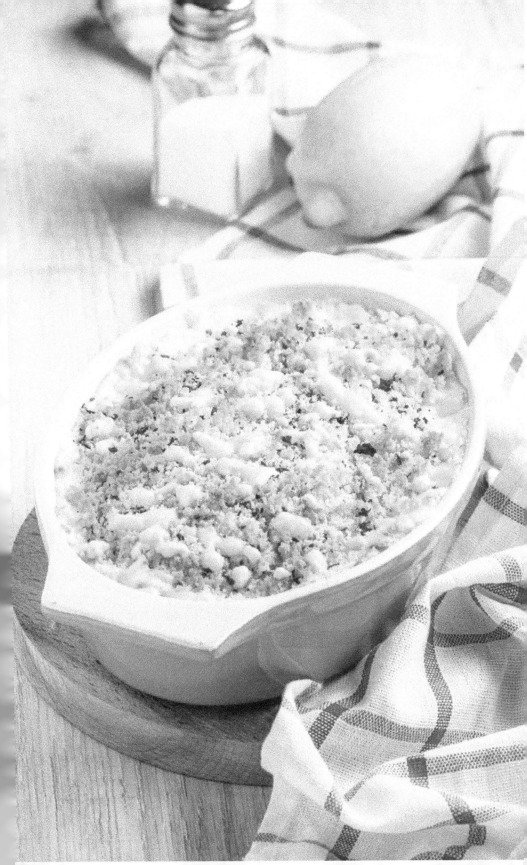

34. Parmesan Sweet Potato Casserole

Preparation Time: 15 minutes

Cooking Time: 35 minutes

Servings: 2

Ingredients:

- 2 sweet potatoes, peeled

- ½ yellow onion, sliced

- ½ cup cream

- ¼ cup spinach

- 2 oz. Parmesan cheese, shredded

- ½ teaspoon salt

- 1 tomato

- teaspoon olive oil

Directions:

1. Preheat the air fryer to 390 °F.

2. Chop the sweet potatoes, the tomato, and the spinach.

3. Spray the air fryer tray with the olive oil.

4. Then, place on a layer of the chopped sweet potato, a layer of the sliced onion, and sprinkle them with the chopped spinach and tomatoes.

5. Season with the salt and the shredded cheese, then pour the cream.

6. Cook for 35 minutes and then serve.

Nutrition: Calories 93, Fat 1,8, Fiber 3,4, Carbs 20,3, Protein 1,8.

35. Roasted Squash Puree

Preparation Time: 20 minutes

Cooking Time: 6 hours

Servings: 8

Ingredients:

- 1 (3-pound) butternut squash, peeled, seeded, and cut into 1- inch pieces

- 3 (1-pound) acorn squash, peeled, seeded, and cut into 1-inch pieces

- 2 onions, chopped

- 3 garlic cloves, minced

- 2 tablespoons olive oil

- 1 teaspoon dried marjoram leaves

- ½ teaspoon of salt

- 1/8 teaspoon of freshly ground black pepper

Directions:

1. In a 6-quart slow cooker, mix all of the ingredients.

2. Cover the pot with the lid and cook on low for 6 to 7 hours, or until the squash is tender.

3. Finally, mash the squash using a potato masher.

Nutrition: Calories 175, Fat 4, Fiber 3, Carbs 38, Protein 3.

36. Roasted Root Vegetables

Preparation Time: 20 minutes

Cooking Time: 6 hours

Servings: 8

Ingredients:

- 6 carrots, cut into 1-inch chunks

- 2 yellow onions, each cut into 8 wedges

- 2 sweet potatoes, peeled and cut into chunks

- 6 Yukon Gold potatoes, cut into chunks

- 8 whole garlic cloves, peeled

- 4 parsnips, peeled and cut into chunks 3 tablespoons olive oil

- 3 teaspoons of dried thyme leaves

- ½ teaspoon of salt

- 1/8 teaspoon of freshly ground black pepper

Directions:

1. In a 6-quart slow cooker, mix all of the ingredients.

2. Cover and cook on low for 6 to 8 hours, or until the vegetables are tender.

3. Serve and enjoy!

Nutrition: Calories 214, Fat 5, Fiber 6, Carbs 40, Protein 4.

37.   Sabich Sandwich

Preparation Time: 5 minutes

Cooking Time: 15 minutes

Servings: 2

Ingredients:

- 2 tomatoes

- Olive oil

- ½ lb. eggplant

- ¼ cucumber

- 1 tablespoon lemon

- 1 tablespoon parsley

- ¼ head cabbage

- 2 tablespoons wine vinegar

- 2 pita bread

- ½ cup hummus

- ¼ tahini sauce

- 2 hard-boiled eggs

Directions:

1. In a skillet, fry eggplant slices until they become tender.

2. Into a bowl, add tomatoes, cucumber, parsley, lemon juice, and season salad.

3. In another bowl, toss cabbage with vinegar.

4. In each pita pocket add hummus, eggplant, and drizzle tahini sauce.

5. Top with eggs and tahini sauce.

Nutrition: Calories 269, Fat 14, Fiber 2, Carbs 2, Protein 7.

38.   Shakshuka

Preparation Time: 10 minutes

Cooking Time: 30 minutes

Servings: 1
Ingredients:

- 1 tablespoon of chopped parsley

- 1 teaspoon of Extra virgin olive oil

- 1 teaspoon of paprika

- ½ cup of red onion finely chopped

- 30g. Kale (stems removed and roughly chopped)

- 1 garlic clove finely chopped

- 30g celery finely chopped

- 1 bird's eye chili finely chopped

- 1 teaspoon of ground turmeric

- 1 teaspoon of ground cumin

- 2 cups of tinned chopped tomatoes

- 2 medium eggs

Directions:

1. In a frying pan add the oil and heat over medium-low heat. Then, add the chili, spices, celery, garlic, and onions and fry for about 2 minutes.

2. Add the tomatoes, then allow the sauce to simmer gently for about 20 minutes and stirring frequently.

3. Add the kale to the pot and cook for another five minutes. (if the sauce gets too thick, add a little water).

4. Stir in the parsley once the sauce becomes nicely creamy.

5. Create two little wells in the sauce, then break each egg into the wells. Reduce the heat to the lowest, cover the pan with its lid and allow the eggs to cook for about 10 minutes (if you want the yolks to be firm, cook for another 4 minutes).

6. Serve immediately.

Nutrition: Calories 657, Fat 4, Carbs 6, Protein 87.

39. Spicy Zucchini Slices

Preparation Time: 10 minutes

Cooking Time: 6 minutes

Servings: 2

Ingredients:

- 1 teaspoon of cornstarch

- 1 zucchini

- ½ teaspoon of chili flakes

- 1 tablespoon of flour

- 1 egg

- ¼ teaspoon salt

Directions:

1. 1.Preheat the air fryer to 400 °F.

2. Slice the zucchini and sprinkle with the chili flakes and salt.

3. Into a bowl, crack the egg into the bowl and whisk it.

4. In a dish, combine cornstarch with the flour and stir it.

5. Dip the zucchini slices in the whisked egg and then in the cornstarch mixture.

6. Place the zucchini slices in the air fryer tray, and cook them for four minutes. After this, flip the slices to the other side and cook for 2 minutes more.

7. Serve the zucchini slices hot.

Nutrition: Calories 67, Fat 2,4, Fiber 1,2, Carbs 7,7, Protein 4,4.

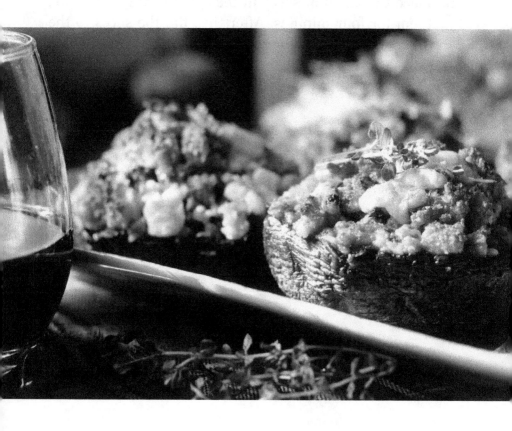

40.   Stuffed Mushrooms

Preparation Time: 7 minutes

Cooking Time: 10 minutes

Servings: 1
Ingredients:

- ½ rashers bacon, diced

- ½ onion, diced

- ½ bell pepper, diced

- ½ small carrot, diced

- 2 medium-size mushrooms (separate the caps and stalks)

- ¼ cup shredded cheddar plus extra for to top

- ¼ cup sour cream

Directions:
1. Preheat the air fryer to 400°C.

2. Chop the mushrooms stalks finely and fry them up with the bacon, onion, pepper, and carrot at 350 ° for 8 minutes.

3. When the veggies are tender, stir in the sour cream and the cheese and keep on the heat until the cheese has melted, and everything is mixed nicely.

---

4. Heap a plop of filling on each mushroom and top with a little extra cheese.

5. Place in the fryer basket and cook them for some minutes. Then serve hot and enjoy!

Nutrition: Calories 285, Fat 20,5, Protein 8,6.

CPSIA information can be obtained
at www.ICGtesting.com
Printed in the USA
BVHW061921220321
603177BV00010B/964

9 781914 105548